Seven Day Ketogenic Diet Meal Plan and Menu

This book contains a comprehensive meal plan for the ketogenic (a high-fat, low-carbohydrate) diet. It discusses the advantages, how to begin, what to eat, what not to eat, and a sample ketogenic diet plan and menu for one week.

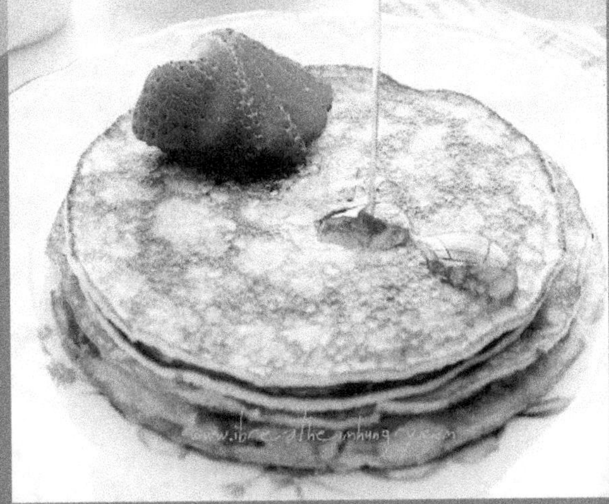

Jane White

COPYWRITE PAGE

Contents

INTRODUCTION

This book contains a comprehensive meal plan for the ketogenic (a high-fat, low-carbohydrate) diet. It discusses the advantages, how to begin, what to eat, what not to eat, and a sample ketogenic diet plan and menu for one week.

Author Jane White was overweight, and as a result became fatigued and depressed. After some times, she came across the ketogenic diet and was surprised that the excess fats she had accumulated melted away and her illness disappears. In this unique, reader-friendly book, Jane shares firsthand experience and practical ideas on how to manage the transition to ketogenic diet.

In contrast to many other books that discuss ketogenic diet, Jane white aggregated ketogenic diet plan with spicy recipes to kick start the keto lifestyle. Jane identifies simple yet nourishing diets.

Features

- Discover the benefits of ketogenic diet
- Detailed information on the nutritional fact of each diet
- Over 100 mouthwatering easy-to-follow recipes
- Explanatory overview that explains the ketogenic diet

Get rid of excess weight with Jane White's 7-day ketogenic diet plan.

CHAPTER ONE

This piece contains a comprehensive meal plan for the ketogenic (a high-fat, low-carbohydrate) diet. Its advantages, how to begin, what to eat, what not to eat, and a sample ketogenic diet plan and menu for one week.

You've most likely heard about the low carbohydrate diets, high fat diet that's so trendy among actors and models, and with good reason: low diets offer appropriate nourishment with complete foods, while charging your body to burn fat for fuel. This is a huge way to be, as it makes fat loss principally effortless! But where does this "ketogenic" word come from, and how does it fit into the picture?

Well, ketogenic is derived from the word 'ketosis', which is a condition in which your body breaks down or metabolizes fat molecules into ketones to provide energy. This state is accomplished through very low carbohydrate intake and higher than normal intake of fat. The "usual" state of the body's metabolism is called 'glycolysis', a process that burns carbohydrates for energy. The truth is that when your body is in carbohydrate-burning mode, it will use all available carbohydrates for energy before touching stored fat. In ketosis, your body is primed to burn fat, and this is great news for anyone who is trying to get trim and slim.

Advantages of Ketosis

By cutting carbohydrate intake significantly, we can hugely reduce insulin resistance, the antecedent to type 2 diabetes. Addition, low carbohydrate diets, alongside exercise, can be very efficient in alleviating the symptoms and development of type 2 diabetes. Furthermore, ketosis itself is appetite-suppressing, which means your hunger will, by nature, check itself, raising your caloric deficit and making you lose fat even faster

Getting Started

Ketosis takes a little time to get into – about 2 weeks of low carbohydrate eating is required for the initial adjustment. During this moment, there will be bouts of lethargy, exhaustion, headaches, and some gastrointestinal problems as you adapt, often referred to as 'keto flu'. Proper intake of electrolytes will correct most of these issues. Additionally, the 'diet' part of this ketogenic meal plan – that is, the caloric constraint – shouldn't be anxious about. Weight loss will come as your body controls appetite as it the addiction to sugar and processed food lessens, so restricting calories during the first two weeks isn't recommended.

The meal plan is intended to ensure you get three (3) balanced, healthy meals a day that tackle fiber, satiation, and sufficient protein intake. The best part of a ketogenic diet is the fact that it spares muscle loss, where a carbohydrate-based diet doesn't. Weight lost in a high carbohydrate, calorie-restricted diet will frequently come both from muscle and fat, while with keto, you can burn fat without giving up muscle. This is referred to frequently as 'body recomposition' and leaves you with a much preferred physique following weight loss.

Additional Points of Interest

Ketogenic diets regularly create a major loss of water during the first phases. This is because carbohydrates are converted to glycogen in the body, which is stored in water within the muscles and liver. As you exhaust stored glycogen, your body washes out this water. This is an enormous part of the early weight loss during the opening few weeks of ketosis. While speedy fat loss does occur at first, a lot of water weight is often lost as well, but this is of great benefit as it often results in both weight loss with a reduction of bloating, allowing clothes to fit better.

Recommended Foods on a Ketogenic Diet

- ❖ **Meat:** Goat, lamb, beef, turkey, pork, chicken, and veal.
- ❖ **Fish:** Trout, catfish, Salmon, sardines, haddock, tuna, and many others.
- ❖ **Fruits:** Blueberries, strawberries, avocado, and raspberries.
- ❖ **Vegetables:** Asparagus, Broccoli, Brussels, cucumbers, sprouts, and many others.
- ❖ **Nuts and Seeds:** Walnuts, Almonds, sunflower, sesame, pumpkin etc.
- ❖ **Dairy Products:** Greek yogurt, cheese, heavy cream, and sour cream.
- ❖ **Fats and Oils:** Flaxseed oil, peanut butter, sesame oil, olive oil, butter, and almond oil.

Foods to Avoid on a Ketogenic Diet

- ❖ **Grains:** Oats, wheat, barley, corn, and rye. This includes pastas and breads.
- ❖ **Artificial Sweeteners**: Equal, Sucralose, Acesulfame, Saccharin, Splenda, etc.
- ❖ **Processed Foods:** Don't eat any food that contains carrageenan.
- ❖ **"Low-fat" products:** Gluten, Atkins products, diet soda, drinks, etc.

CHAPTER TWO

Healthfully go into Ketosis with This scrumptious 7-Day "Ketogenic" Meal Plan and list of options.

Day One

(Total: 1650 calories, 130g fat, 15g net carbs, 88g protein)

Breakfast

- ✓ Three Inch Square Sausage and Spinach Frittata (See Table 1 and Figure 1)
- ✓ Coffee with two Tbsp. Heavy Cream (See Table 2)

Three Inch Square, Sausage and Spinach Frittata

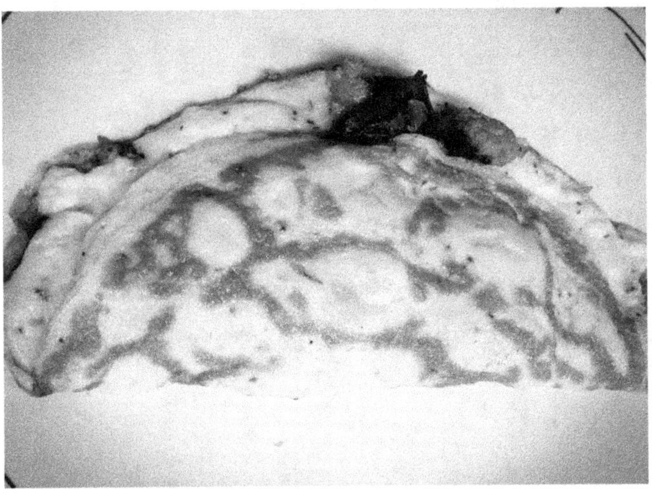

Figure1: *Sausage, Spinach and Feta Frittata – Low carbohydrate & Gluten Free*

Table 1. Nutritional facts for Three Inch Square Sausage & Spinach Frittata

Nutrition Facts

Serving size	1 1 (59g)

Amount Per Serving

Calories 140

% Daily Value*

Total Fat 21g	**27%**
Saturated Fat 6g	**30%**
Trans Fat 0g	
Cholesterol 385mg	**128%**
Sodium 540mg	**24%**
Total Carbohydrate 5g	**2%**
Dietary Fiber 1g	**4%**
Total Sugars 0g	
Includes 0g Added Sugars	**0%**
Protein 25g	**50%**
Vitamin D 0mcg	0%
Calcium 0mg	0%
Iron 0mg	0%
Potassium 0mg	0%

*The % Daily Value (DV) tells you how much a nutrient in a serving of food contributes to a daily diet. 2,000 calories a day is used for general nutrition advice.

Recipes: Sausage, Spinach, and Feta Frittata

Ingredients

- Olive oil (2 tablespoons)
- Medium sweet (2 pieces) or about 10 oz. hot Italian sausages.
- 1 package iced chopped spinach, melted according to package advice.
- roasted red peppers (2 ounces) cut into strips
- Eggs lightly beaten (10 pcs)
- Shredded Parmesan (1/2 cup, 2 oz.)

Preparation

1. Preheat oven to about 400°F. In a big nonstick, oven-proof skillet, warm the olive oil over medium-to-high heat. Note: If the skillet is not oven-proof, wrap up handles in a twofold layer of foil.) Take out sausages from case and crush the meat into skillet. Cook, stir and break up big pieces till there are no traces of pink. This is done in about 10 minutes.
2. Squash as much fluid as possible from the spinach. Pour surplus fat from the skillet; include spinach & red peppers. Cook, stir well, and scrap up any cooked bit on the bottom of the skillet.
3. Pour the eggs into the skillet and stir well to mix with the spinach-sausage mixture. Stop stirring at this point and boil over average heat. Lift the edges of frittata with a spatula to allow lightly- or uncooked eggs move underneath. Cook for about 3 minutes until everything looks set.
4. Spray the Parmesan on top and then transfer the skillet to oven. Bake naked, until frittata is winded and slightly browned at the top, this takes about 8 to 10 minutes. Lift frittata about the edges of skillet and tenderly shake the pan to get loosen. Slip out of pan and onto a cutting board or plank and then cut into blocks. Serve the meal hot or at a room temperature.

Coffee with Two Tablespoon Heavy Cream

Table 2. Nutritional facts for **Coffee with two Tbsp. Heavy Cream**

Nutrition Facts

Serving size

Amount Per Serving

Calories 120

	% Daily Value*
Total Fat 12g	15%
Saturated Fat 0g	0%
Trans Fat 0g	
Sodium 0mg	0%
Total Carbohydrate 1g	0%
Dietary Fiber 0g	0%
Total Sugars 0g	
Includes 0g Added Sugars	0%
Protein 0g	0%

Not a significant source of cholesterol, vitamin D, calcium, iron, and potassium

*The % Daily Value (DV) tells you how much a nutrient in a serving of food contributes to a daily diet. 2,000 calories a day is used for general nutrition advice.

✓ **Half Hass Avocado with Slight Salt & Pepper**

Table 3. Nutritional facts for Half Hass Avocado with Slight Salt & Pepper

Nutrition Facts

Serving size

Amount Per Serving

Calories   **110**

	% Daily Value*
Total Fat 11g	14%
Saturated Fat 0g	0%
Trans Fat 0g	
Sodium 0mg	0%
Total Carbohydrate 1g	0%
Dietary Fiber 0g	0%
Total Sugars 0g	
Includes 0g Added Sugars	0%
Protein 1g	2%

Not a significant source of cholesterol, vitamin D, calcium, iron, and potassium

*The % Daily Value (DV) tells you how much a nutrient in a serving of food contributes to a daily diet. 2,000 calories a day is used for general nutrition advice.

- ✓ Half Cup Simple Egg Salad (See Table 4 and Figure 2)
- ✓ Four (4) Romaine Lettuce Leaves (See Table 5)
- ✓ Two (2) Cooked Sliced Bacon (See Table 6)

Half (½) Cup Simple Egg Salad

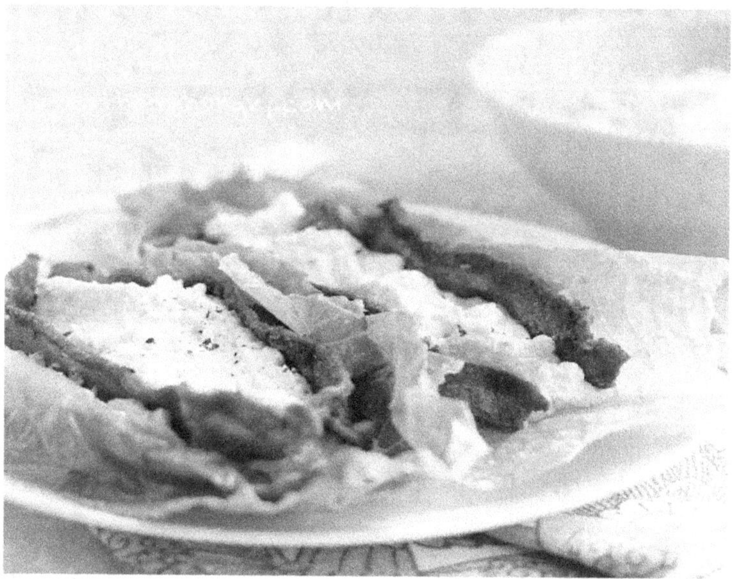

Fig. 2: *Easy-Low Carbohydrate Egg Salad*

Table 4. Nutritional facts for Easy-Low Carbohydrate Egg Salad

Nutrition Facts

Serving size	**1 1 (59g)**

Amount Per Serving

Calories 300

% Daily Value*

Total Fat 29g	**37%**
Saturated Fat 0g	**0%**
Trans Fat 0g	
Cholesterol 0mg	**0%**
Sodium 0mg	**0%**
Total Carbohydrate 2g	**1%**
Dietary Fiber 0g	**1%**
Total Sugars 1g	
Includes 0g Added Sugars	**0%**
Protein 9g	**17%**
Vitamin D 0mcg	**0%**
Calcium 0mg	**0%**
Iron 0mg	**0%**
Potassium 0mg	**0%**

*The % Daily Value (DV) tells you how much a nutrient in a serving of food contributes to a daily diet. 2,000 calories a day is used for general nutrition advice.

Recipes: Easy-Low Carbohydrate Egg Salad

Preparation Time: 10 min.

Cook Time: 7 min.

Total Time: 17 min.

Servings: 4

Calories: 305 kcal

Ingredients

- Six (6) hard-boiled eggs.
- Half cup full mayonnaise fat.
- Half – One tbsp. curry powder (to enhance taste).

Instructions

1. To prepare the boiled eggs, put the eggs in a pan and cover it with iced water.
2. Put on the heat and once the water starts to boil, wait for 7 minutes.
3. Sap and cover with iced water to prevent them from further cooking.
4. Once it is cool, unwrap and cut the eggs into little pieces.
5. Blend the eggs, curry powder, and mayonnaise.
6. Dish up with sliced fresh parsley.

Four (4) Romaine Lettuce Leaves

Table 5. Nutritional facts for Four (4) Romaine Lettuce Leaves

Nutrition Facts

Serving size

Amount Per Serving

Calories 5

	% Daily Value*
Total Fat 0g	**0%**
Saturated Fat 0g	**0%**
Trans Fat 0g	
Sodium 0mg	**0%**
Total Carbohydrate 0g	**0%**
Dietary Fiber 0g	**0%**
Total Sugars 0g	
Includes 0g Added Sugars	**0%**
Protein 0g	**0%**

Not a significant source of cholesterol, vitamin D, calcium, iron, and potassium

*The % Daily Value (DV) tells you how much a nutrient in a serving of food contributes to a daily diet. 2,000 calories a day is used for general nutrition advice.

Two (2) Cooked Sliced Bacon

Table 6. Nutritional Facts for Two (2) Cooked Sliced Bacon

Nutrition Facts

Serving size

Amount Per Serving

Calories 90

	% Daily Value*
Total Fat 7g	**9%**
Saturated Fat 0g	**0%**
Trans Fat 0g	
Sodium 0mg	**0%**
Total Carbohydrate 0g	**0%**
Dietary Fiber 0g	**0%**
Total Sugars 0g	
Includes 0g Added Sugars	**0%**
Protein 6g	**12%**

Not a significant source of cholesterol, vitamin D, calcium, iron, and potassium

*The % Daily Value (DV) tells you how much a nutrient in a serving of food contributes to a daily diet. 2,000 calories a day is used for general nutrition advice.

Snack

   ✓ **Raw Almonds**

Table 7. Nutritional Facts for Raw Almonds

Nutrition Facts

Serving size

Amount Per Serving

Calories 170

	% Daily Value*
Total Fat 15g	**19%**
Saturated Fat 0g	**0%**
Trans Fat 0g	
Sodium 0mg	**0%**
Total Carbohydrate 2g	**1%**
Dietary Fiber 0g	**0%**
Total Sugars 0g	
Includes 0g Added Sugars	**0%**
Protein 6g	**12%**

Not a significant source of cholesterol, vitamin D, calcium, iron, and potassium

*The % Daily Value (DV) tells you how much a nutrient in a serving of food contributes to a daily diet. 2,000 calories a day is used for general nutrition advice.

Dinner

- ✓ Six (6) oz rotisserie chicken (See Table 8).

- ✓ Three-quarter (3/4) Cup Easy Cauliflower Gratin (See Table 9 and Figure 3).

- ✓ Two (2) Cups chopped romaine-lettuce (See Table 10)

- ✓ Two (2) Tablespoon Caesar-Salad Dressing (sugar free) (See Table 11).

Six (6) Oz Rotisserie Chicken

Table 8. Nutritional facts for six (6) Oz Rotisserie Chicken

Nutrition Facts

Serving size

Amount Per Serving

Calories 280

	% Daily Value*
Total Fat 11g	14%
Saturated Fat 0g	0%
Trans Fat 0g	
Sodium 0mg	0%
Total Carbohydrate 0g	0%
Dietary Fiber 0g	0%
Total Sugars 0g	
Includes 0g Added Sugars	0%
Protein 42g	84%

Not a significant source of cholesterol, vitamin D, calcium, iron, and potassium

*The % Daily Value (DV) tells you how much a nutrient in a serving of food contributes to a daily diet. 2,000 calories a day is used for general nutrition advice.

Three-Quarter (3/4) Cup Easy-Cauliflower Gratin

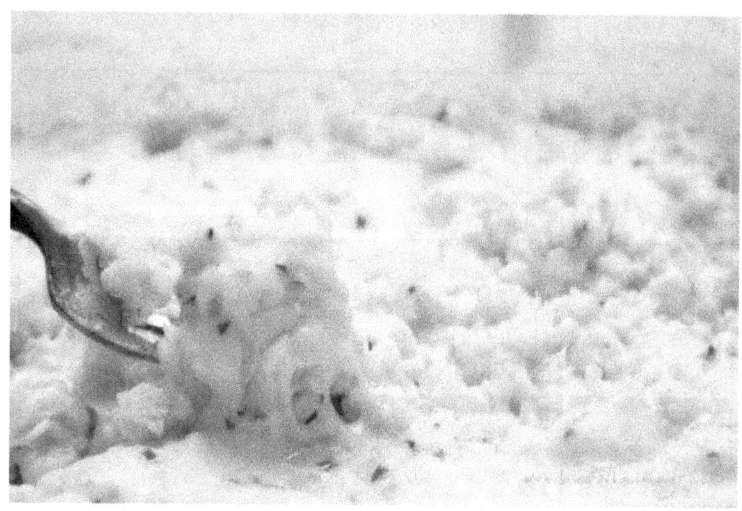

Fig. 3: *Easy Cheesy-Cauliflower Gratin Recipe (Low Carbohydrate and Gluten-Free)*

Table 9. Nutritional Facts for Easy Cheesy Cauliflower Gratin Recipe (Low Carbohydrate and Gluten-Free)

Nutrition Facts

Serving size

Amount Per Serving

Calories 30

	% Daily Value*
Total Fat 2g	**3%**
Saturated Fat 1.1g	**6%**
Trans Fat 0g	
Cholesterol 25mg	**9%**
Sodium 45mg	**2%**
Total Carbohydrate 1g	**0%**
Dietary Fiber < 1g	**2%**
Total Sugars < 1g	
Includes 0g Added Sugars	**0%**
Protein 2g	**5%**
Vitamin D 0mcg	**0%**
Calcium 0mg	**0%**
Iron 0mg	**0%**
Potassium 0mg	**0%**

*The % Daily Value (DV) tells you how much a nutrient in a serving of food contributes to a daily diet. 2,000 calories a day is used for general nutrition advice.

Recipe for making Easy Cheesy Cauliflower-Gratin Recipe

Prep Time: 10 mins

Cook Time: 40 mins

Total Time: 50 mins

These Easy-Cheesy Cauliflower tots are gluten-free, low carbohydrate, and absolutely delicious! These tots are the ideal modest healthy snack that will satisfy even the most selective eaters.

Servings: 30

Calories: 30 kcal

Ingredients

- Four (4) cups riced cauliflower
- One (1) cup shredded cheddar cheese
- One (1) cup shredded mozzarella cheese
- Three (3) minced cloves garlic.
- Half (1/2) tbsp. Italian seasoning.
- Four (4) eggs.
- Pepper and salt to enhance taste.

Instructions

1. Pre-heat your oven to about 425°F. set up a huge baking sheet using parchment paper.
2. Slice the cauliflower into little florets and include them in your food processor. Pound a little times till the cauliflower look like rice.
3. Put the cauliflower in a microwave-like container and cover up with lid. Microwave for about 10 minutes. Put the micro-waved cauliflower in a big bowl and allow cooling for about 5 minutes.
4. Add the garlic, cheeses, Italian seasoning, eggs, salt, and pepper to the cauliflower and blend the whole thing together until fully incorporated.
5. Get about one tablespoon of the cauliflower blend and shape it into little tots, and then put them on the arranged baking sheet. Do this again with all the remaining cauliflower.
6. Bake for 30 minutes and/or until it becomes golden brown. Generally, I put them under the broiler for some minutes to obtain the pleasant golden color.
7. Dish up with sour cream, pizza sauce, or dairy farm dip ketchup.

Recipe Notes

If you do not have a food processor, you could grate the uncooked cauliflower using the uncouth surface of the grater.

If you don't have a microwave, I would recommend that you first cook the cauliflower either in your own oven or on the stove before ricing it. The easiest method would be steaming followed by ricing.

Please note that the nutritional information provided herein is a rough estimation and may differ significantly based on products utilized.

Two (2) Cups Chopped-Romaine Lettuce

Table 10. Nutritional facts for Two (2) Cups Chopped-Romaine Lettuce

Nutrition Facts

Serving size

Amount Per Serving

Calories 15

	% Daily Value*
Total Fat 0g	0%
Saturated Fat 0g	0%
Trans Fat 0g	
Sodium 0mg	0%
Total Carbohydrate 1g	0%
Dietary Fiber 0g	0%
Total Sugars 0g	
Includes 0g Added Sugars	0%
Protein 1g	2%

Not a significant source of cholesterol, vitamin D, calcium, iron, and potassium

*The % Daily Value (DV) tells you how much a nutrient in a serving of food contributes to a daily diet. 2,000 calories a day is used for general nutrition advice.

Two (2) Tablespoon Caesar-Salad Dressing (Sugar Free)

Table 11. Nutritional facts for Two (2) Tablespoon Caesar-Salad Dressing

Nutrition Facts

Serving size

Amount Per Serving

Calories 170

% Daily Value*

Total Fat 18g	23%
Saturated Fat 0g	0%
Trans Fat 0g	
Sodium 0mg	0%
Total Carbohydrate 2g	1%
Dietary Fiber 0g	0%
Total Sugars 0g	
Includes 0g Added Sugars	0%
Protein 1g	2%

Not a significant source of cholesterol, vitamin D, calcium, iron, and potassium

*The % Daily Value (DV) tells you how much a nutrient in a serving of food contributes to a daily diet. 2,000 calories a day is used for general nutrition advice.

- ✓ **Two (2) squares Lindt 90 Percent Chocolate**

Table 12. Nutritional Facts for Two (2) squares Lindt 90 Percent Chocolate

Nutrition Facts

Serving size

Amount Per Serving

Calories 100

	% Daily Value*
Total Fat 9g	12%
Saturated Fat 0g	0%
Trans Fat 0g	
Sodium 0mg	0%
Total Carbohydrate 3g	1%
Dietary Fiber 0g	0%
Total Sugars 0g	
Includes 0g Added Sugars	0%
Protein 3g	6%

Not a significant source of cholesterol, vitamin D, calcium, iron, and potassium

*The % Daily Value (DV) tells you how much a nutrient in a serving of food contributes to a daily diet. 2,000 calories a day is used for general nutrition advice.

Day Two

(Totals: 1640 calories, 130g fat, 19g net carbs, 90g protein)

Breakfast

- ✓ Three (3) Inch-square Sausage & Spinach Frittata (See Table 1 and Figure 1)

- ✓ Coffee with two (2) Tablespoon Heavy Cream (See Table 2)

✓ **Five (5) Sticks of Celery with Two (2) Tablespoon Almond Butter**

Table 13. Nutritional facts for Five (5) sticks of celery with (2) Tbsp. Almond Butter

Nutrition Facts

Serving size

Amount Per Serving

Calories 200

% Daily Value*

Total Fat 16g	**21%**
Saturated Fat 0g	**0%**
Trans Fat 0g	
Sodium 0mg	**0%**
Total Carbohydrate 2g	**1%**
Dietary Fiber 0g	**0%**
Total Sugars 0g	
Includes 0g Added Sugars	**0%**
Protein 7g	**14%**

Not a significant source of cholesterol, vitamin D, calcium, iron, and potassium

*The % Daily Value (DV) tells you how much a nutrient in a serving of food contributes to a daily diet. 2,000 calories a day is used for general nutrition advice.

Lunch

- ✓ **2 cups chopped romaine lettuce (See Table 10)**

- ✓ **2 Tbsp Caesar Salad Dressing (sugar free) (See Table 11)**

- ✓ **1 cup chopped leftover chicken (See Table 14)**

One (1) Cup Chopped-Leftover Chicken

Table 14. Nutritional facts for one (1) Cup Chopped-Leftover Chicken

Nutrition Facts

Serving size

Amount Per Serving

Calories 280

% Daily Value*

Total Fat 11g	**14%**
Saturated Fat 0g	**0%**
Trans Fat 0g	
Sodium 0mg	**0%**
Total Carbohydrate 0g	**0%**
Dietary Fiber 0g	**0%**
Total Sugars 0g	
Includes 0g Added Sugars	**0%**
Protein 42g	**84%**

Not a significant source of cholesterol, vitamin D, calcium, iron, and potassium

*The % Daily Value (DV) tells you how much a nutrient in a serving of food contributes to a daily diet. 2,000 calories a day is used for general nutrition advice.

✓ **Half Hass Avocado with Slight Salt & Pepper (See Table 15)**

Table 15. Nutritional facts for Half Hass Avocado with Slight Salt & Pepper

Nutrition Facts

Serving size

Amount Per Serving

Calories 110

	% Daily Value*
Total Fat 11g	14%
Saturated Fat 0g	0%
Trans Fat 0g	
Sodium 0mg	0%
Total Carbohydrate 1g	0%
Dietary Fiber 0g	0%
Total Sugars 0g	
Includes 0g Added Sugars	0%
Protein 1g	2%

Not a significant source of cholesterol, vitamin D, calcium, iron, and potassium

*The % Daily Value (DV) tells you how much a nutrient in a serving of food contributes to a daily diet. 2,000 calories a day is used for general nutrition advice.

Dinner

- ✓ **One (1) Italian sausage link – cooked & sliced (See Table 16)**

- ✓ **One (1) cup broccoli – cooked (See Table 17)**

- ✓ **One (1) Tablespoon butter (See Table 18)**

- ✓ **Two (2) Tablespoon parmesan cheese – grated (See Table 19)**

One (1) Italian sausage link – cooked & sliced

Table 16. Nutritional facts for One (1) Italian sausage link – cooked & sliced

Nutrition Facts

Serving size

Amount Per Serving

Calories 230

% Daily Value*

Total Fat 18g	**23%**
Saturated Fat 0g	**0%**
Trans Fat 0g	
Sodium 0mg	**0%**
Total Carbohydrate 1g	**0%**
Dietary Fiber 0g	**0%**
Total Sugars 0g	
Includes 0g Added Sugars	**0%**
Protein 13g	**26%**

Not a significant source of cholesterol, vitamin D, calcium, iron, and potassium

*The % Daily Value (DV) tells you how much a nutrient in a serving of food contributes to a daily diet. 2,000 calories a day is used for general nutrition advice.

One (1) cup broccoli – cooked

Table 17. Nutritional facts for One (1) cup broccoli – cooked

Nutrition Facts

Serving size

Amount Per Serving

Calories 60

	% Daily Value*
Total Fat 0g	0%
Saturated Fat 0g	0%
Trans Fat 0g	
Sodium 0mg	0%
Total Carbohydrate 6g	2%
Dietary Fiber 0g	0%
Total Sugars 0g	
Includes 0g Added Sugars	0%
Protein 4g	8%

Not a significant source of cholesterol, vitamin D, calcium, iron, and potassium

*The % Daily Value (DV) tells you how much a nutrient in a serving of food contributes to a daily diet. 2,000 calories a day is used for general nutrition advice.

One (1) Tablespoon butter

Table 18. Nutritional facts for One (1) Tablespoon butter

Nutrition Facts

Serving size

Amount Per Serving

Calories 100

	% Daily Value*
Total Fat 12g	**15%**
Saturated Fat 0g	**0%**
Trans Fat 0g	
Sodium 0mg	**0%**
Total Carbohydrate 0g	**0%**
Dietary Fiber 0g	**0%**
Total Sugars 0g	
Includes 0g Added Sugars	**0%**
Protein 0g	**0%**

Not a significant source of cholesterol, vitamin D, calcium, iron, and potassium

*The % Daily Value (DV) tells you how much a nutrient in a serving of food contributes to a daily diet. 2,000 calories a day is used for general nutrition advice.

Two (2) Tablespoon parmesan cheese – grated

Table 19. Nutritional facts for Two (2) Tablespoon parmesan cheese – grated

Nutrition Facts

Serving size

Amount Per Serving

Calories 40

% Daily Value*

Total Fat 3g	**4%**
Saturated Fat 0g	**0%**
Trans Fat 0g	
Sodium 0mg	**0%**
Total Carbohydrate 0g	**0%**
Dietary Fiber 0g	**0%**
Total Sugars 0g	
Includes 0g Added Sugars	**0%**
Protein 4g	**8%**

Not a significant source of cholesterol, vitamin D, calcium, iron, and potassium

*The % Daily Value (DV) tells you how much a nutrient in a serving of food contributes to a daily diet. 2,000 calories a day is used for general nutrition advice.

Dessert

- ✓ **Two (2) squares Lindt 90 Percent Chocolate (See Table 12)**

Day Three

(Totals: 1510 calories, 120g fat, 20g net carbs, 80g protein)

Breakfast

- ✓ **Two (2) Cream-Cheese Pancakes (See Table 20 and figure 4)**

- ✓ **Two (2) Pieces Bacon – Cooked (See Table 21)**

- ✓ **Coffee with two Tbsp. Heavy Cream (See Table 2)**

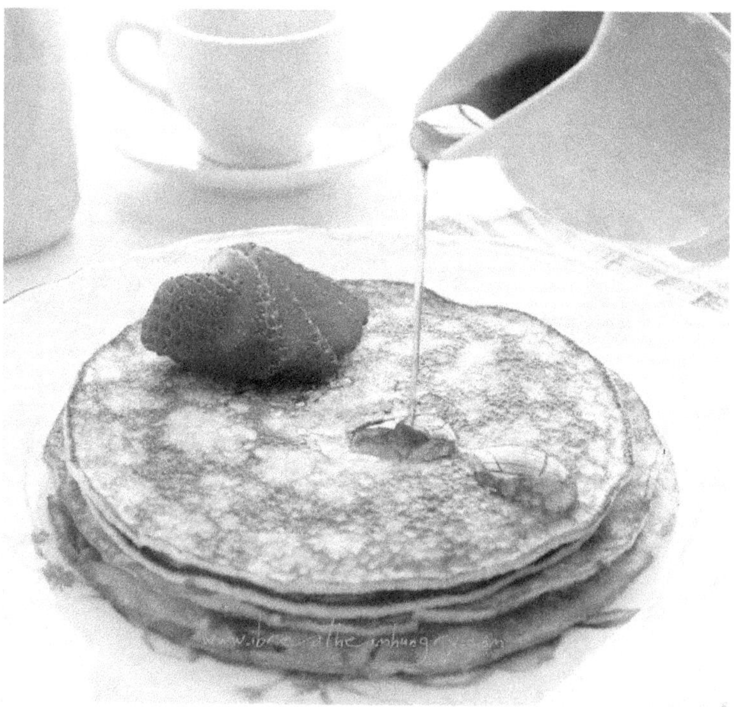

Fig. 4: *Cream-Cheese Pancakes (Low Carbohydate and Gluten-Free)*

Cream-Cheese Pancakes (Low Carbohydrate &Gluten Free)

Table 20. Nutritional facts for Cream-Cheese Pancakes (Low Carbohydrate & Gluten Free)

Nutrition Facts

Serving size

Amount Per Serving

Calories 150

	% Daily Value*
Total Fat 13g	16%
Saturated Fat 6.7g	34%
Trans Fat 0g	
Cholesterol 185mg	62%
Sodium 130mg	6%
Total Carbohydrate 2g	1%
Dietary Fiber < 1g	3%
Total Sugars 0g	
Includes 0g Added Sugars	0%
Protein 7g	14%
Vitamin D 0mcg	0%
Calcium 0.3mg	0%
Iron 0.5mg	2%
Potassium 86mg	2%

*The % Daily Value (DV) tells you how much a nutrient in a serving of food contributes to a daily diet. 2,000 calories a day is used for general nutrition advice.

Recipe for making Cream-Cheese Pancakes

If you are on a ketogenic diet, you will be keen on this easy-low carbohydrate pancake formula. It can assist you get through initiation or weight loss period.

Preparation Time: 2 min.

Cook Time: 7 min.

Total Time: 9 min.

Servings: 7 people

Calories: 150 kcal

Ingredients

- Six (6) large eggs / 4 duck eggs
- Six (6) ounces cream-cheese
- Fifteen (15) drops vanilla-stevia drops (optional)
- One (1) tablespoon psyllium-husks (whole)

Instructions

1. Put all ingredients in a little blender / food processor and mix together until smooth.
2. Dispense about 3 tbsp. batter onto a hot griddle / big frying pan for every pancake.
3. When top is enclosed in foam and boundaries appear dry, turn over pancakes. Go on with cooking until underside is browned.
4. Take away from griddle. Dish up warm with butter & syrup if needed.

Recipe Notes

Each serving includes about 0.9 gram carbohydrate.

Two (2) Pieces Bacon – Cooked

Table 21. Nutritional facts for Two (2) Pieces Bacon – Cooked

Nutrition Facts

Serving size

Amount Per Serving

Calories 90

% Daily Value*

Total Fat 7g	**9%**
Saturated Fat 0g	**0%**
Trans Fat 0g	
Sodium 0mg	**0%**
Total Carbohydrate 0g	**0%**
Dietary Fiber 0g	**0%**
Total Sugars 0g	
Includes 0g Added Sugars	**0%**
Protein 6g	**12%**

Not a significant source of cholesterol, vitamin D, calcium, iron, and potassium

*The % Daily Value (DV) tells you how much a nutrient in a serving of food contributes to a daily diet. 2,000 calories a day is used for general nutrition advice.

✓ **One (1) cup bone broth**

Table 22. Nutritional facts for One (1) cup bone broth

Nutrition Facts

Serving size

Amount Per Serving

Calories 50

% Daily Value*

Total Fat 1g	**1%**
Saturated Fat 0g	**0%**
Trans Fat 0g	
Sodium 0mg	**0%**
Total Carbohydrate 0g	**0%**
Dietary Fiber 0g	**0%**
Total Sugars 0g	
Includes 0g Added Sugars	**0%**
Protein 1g	**2%**

Not a significant source of cholesterol, vitamin D, calcium, iron, and potassium

*The % Daily Value (DV) tells you how much a nutrient in a serving of food contributes to a daily diet. 2,000 calories a day is used for general nutrition advice.

- ✓ One (1) Italian sausage link – cooked & sliced (See Table 16).

- ✓ Three-quarter (3/4) Cup Easy Cauliflower Gratin (See Table 9 and Figure 3).

- ✓ 1.5 Cup Chili-Spaghetti Squash Casserole (See Table 23 and Figure 5)

- ✓ Two (2) Cups Baby Spinach – Raw (See Table 24)

- ✓ One (1) Tablespoon Ranch-Dressing (sugar free) (See Table 25).

1.5 Cup Chili-Spaghetti Squash Casserole

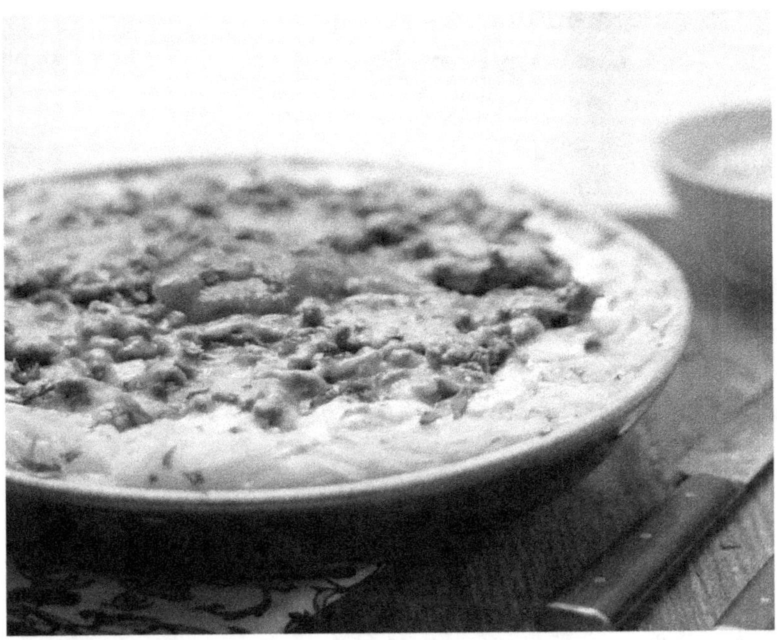

Fig. 5: *Cheesy Chili Spaghetti Squash Casserole – Low Carb and Gluten Free*

Table 23. Nutritional facts for 1.5 Cup Chili-Spaghetti Squash Casserole

Nutrition Facts

Serving size

Amount Per Serving

Calories 190

	% Daily Value*
Total Fat 12g	15%
Saturated Fat 6g	30%
Trans Fat 0g	
Cholesterol 55mg	18%
Sodium 600mg	26%
Total Carbohydrate 7g	3%
Dietary Fiber 1g	4%
Total Sugars 1g	
Includes 0g Added Sugars	0%
Protein 13g	26%
Vitamin D 0mcg	0%
Calcium 75mg	6%
Iron 1.7mg	10%
Potassium 370mg	8%
Vitamin A	8%
Vitamin C	6%

*The % Daily Value (DV) tells you how much a nutrient in a serving of food contributes to a daily diet. 2,000 calories a day is used for general nutrition advice.

Recipe for Making Chili-Spaghetti Squash Casserole

A little carbohydrate & gluten-free casserole formula loaded with chili & cheese on a spaghetti-squash base. Simple and easy to make and it is family friendly!

Serving: 8 persons

Ingredients
For the chili:

- One (1) lb. ground beef – lean (or turkey)
- One (1) teaspoon ground-cumin
- One (1) teaspoon ground coriander
- One (1) tablespoon chopped
- Half (½) teaspoon garlic powder
- One (1) teaspoon dried oregano
- Half (½) prepared salsa
- pepper and salt to enhance taste

For the casserole

- Four (4) cups spaghetti squash – cooked
- Two (2) tbsp. butter – melted
- Three Quarter (¾) cup sour-cream
- 1.75 cup cheddar cheese – shredded
- Sliced cilantro (optional)
- Salsa, sour cream, avocado to serve (optional)

Instructions
For the chili:

1. In an average saucepan brown the meat and season with pepper and salt. Decant any superfluous fat and throw away. Include the remaining of the chili ingredients & cook for about 10 minutes.

For the casserole:

1. In an average bowl mix the cooked spaghetti-quash & thawed butter, toss to coat. Season nicely with pepper and salt to taste.
2. Extend the squash out in a 10 - 15 inch casserole plate. Spray with three-quarter cup of frayed cheese. Extend the sour cream on the cheese coating. Spoon out on the chili & spread it out, leaving a one inch border of spaghetti-squash around the edge. Top with the residual one cup of (shredded) cheese. Bake in a 350°F oven for about 30 min or until well heated. Spray with cilantro & serve with salsa, sour cream, and avocado slices or guacamole as desired.

Two (2) Cups Baby Spinach – Raw

Table 24. Nutritional facts for Two (2) Cups Baby Spinach – Raw

Nutrition Facts

Serving size

Amount Per Serving

Calories 15

	% Daily Value*
Total Fat 0g	**0%**
Saturated Fat 0g	**0%**
Trans Fat 0g	
Sodium 0mg	**0%**
Total Carbohydrate 1g	**0%**
Dietary Fiber 0g	**0%**
Total Sugars 0g	
Includes 0g Added Sugars	**0%**
Protein 2g	**4%**

Not a significant source of cholesterol, vitamin D, calcium, iron, and potassium

*The % Daily Value (DV) tells you how much a nutrient in a serving of food contributes to a daily diet. 2,000 calories a day is used for general nutrition advice.

One (1) Tablespoon Ranch-Dressing (sugar free)

Table 25. Nutritional facts for One (1) Tablespoon Ranch-Dressing

Nutrition Facts

Serving size

Amount Per Serving

Calories 70

	% Daily Value*
Total Fat 7g	9%
Saturated Fat 0g	0%
Trans Fat 0g	
Sodium 0mg	0%
Total Carbohydrate 1g	0%
Dietary Fiber 0g	0%
Total Sugars 0g	
Includes 0g Added Sugars	0%
Protein 0g	0%

Not a significant source of cholesterol, vitamin D, calcium, iron, and potassium

*The % Daily Value (DV) tells you how much a nutrient in a serving of food contributes to a daily diet. 2,000 calories a day is used for general nutrition advice.

Dessert

- ✓ Two (2) squares Lindt 90 Percent Chocolate (See Table 12)

Day Four

(Totals: 1380 calories, 110g fat, 20g net carbs, 70g protein)

Breakfast

- ✓ Three (3) inch square Sausage & Spinach Frittata (See Table 1 and Figure 1)
- ✓ Coffee with (2) two Tablespoon Heavy Cream (See Table 2)

Snack

- ✓ Half (1/2) Hass avocado with light salt & pepper (See Table 15)

Lunch

- ✓ 1.5 cup Chili Spaghetti-Squash Casserole (See Table 23 and Figure 5)

Snack

- ✓ One (1) cup bone-broth (See Table 22)

Dinner

- ✓ Half cup (1/2 cup) Anti-Pasta Salad (See Table 26 and figure 6)
- ✓ Four (4) Sundried Tomato & Feta Meatballs (See Table 27 and figure 7)

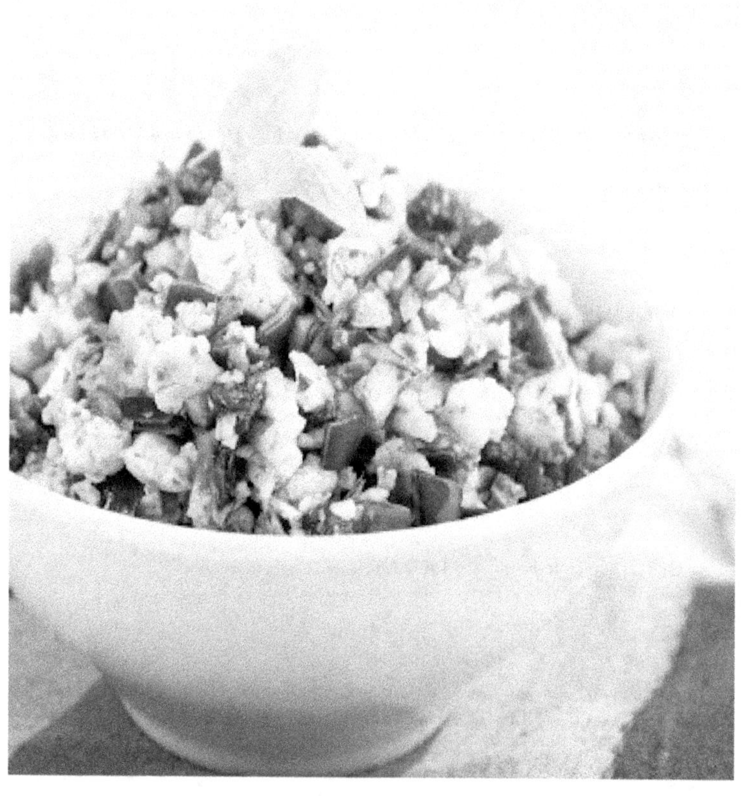

Fig.6: *Anti- Pasta Cauliflower Salad - Low Carbohydrates and Gluten Free*

Table 26. Nutritional facts for Ant-iPasta Cauliflower Salad

Nutrition Facts

Serving size

Amount Per Serving

Calories 100

% Daily Value*

Total Fat 8g	**10%**
Saturated Fat 0g	**0%**
Trans Fat 0g	
Cholesterol 0mg	**0%**
Sodium 0mg	**0%**
Total Carbohydrate 4g	**1%**
Dietary Fiber 0g	**0%**
Total Sugars 0g	
Includes 0g Added Sugars	**0%**
Protein 3g	**6%**
Vitamin D 0mcg	0%
Calcium 0mg	0%
Iron 0mg	0%
Potassium 0mg	0%

*The % Daily Value (DV) tells you how much a nutrient in a serving of food contributes to a daily diet. 2,000 calories a day is used for general nutrition advice.

Recipe for making Anti-Pasta Cauliflower Salad

Type of Recipe: Salad
Cuisine: Pasta salad
Serves: 8.5 cup servings

Constituents

- Two (2) cups of raw chopped cauliflower.
- Half (½) cup of chopped radicchio.
- Half (½) cup of chopped artichoke hearts.
- ⅓ Cup of chopped fresh basil.
- ½ cup of freshly grated parmesan.
- Three (3) Tablespoons of chopped sundried-tomatoes.
- Three (3) Tablespoons of chopped kalamata olives.
- One (1) clove of minced garlic.
- Three (3) Tablespoons of balsamic vinegar.
- Three (3) Tablespoons of 3 extra virgin olive oil.
- Salt & pepper to taste.

Instructions

1. Foremost, cook your lightly sliced cauliflower in the microwave for (5) five minutes. Don't include any liquid or seasoning, just extend it on a microwave and zap it. Let the cauliflower chill while you prepare the other constituents.
2. Mix the radicchio, basil, artichoke hearts, sundried tomatoes, parmesan, olives, and garlic in a medium basin.
3. In a smaller basin, whip together the olive-oil & vinegar, then pour it on the salad. Flip to mix, then season with salt & pepper to taste. It may be served at room temperature / chilled.

Notes

To get the best results, use a high-quality additional virgin olive oil. The artichoke hearts must be crowded in water, not marinated in oil & seasonings.

Also, the sundried tomatoes to be used should be packed in oil so they may be nice and soft - if you use the parched ones, dissolve in some warm water for about 20 min. before use.

Lastly, use a tattered parmesan /asiago, not the coarse grated substance you get from the can.

If you make use of the best worth constituent, it will create an enormous distinction in the flavor.

Do not be anxious by the extended list of ingredient – I assure you that it's worth it!

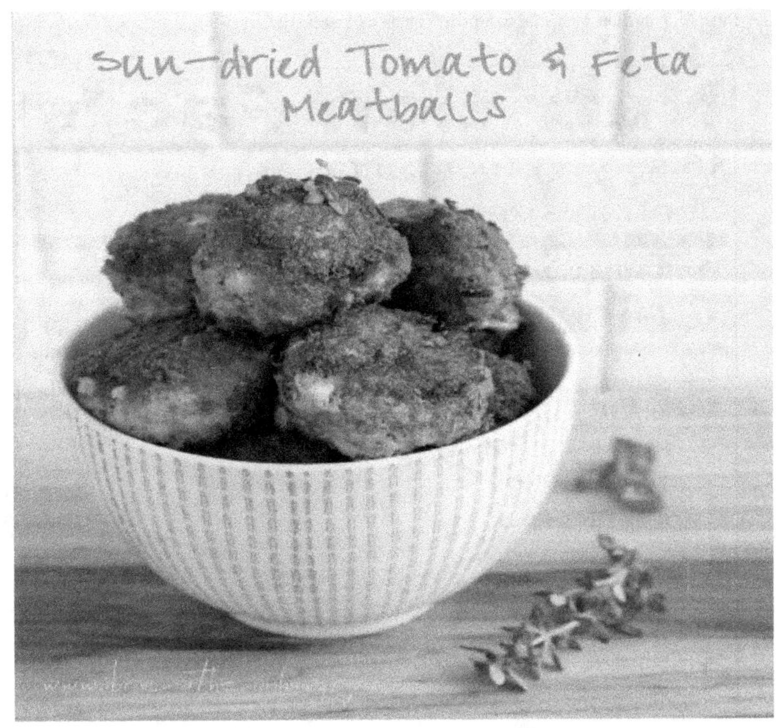

Fig. 7: *Sun-dried Tomato & Feta Meatballs (Low Carbohydrates & Gluten Free)*

Table 27. Nutritional facts for Sun-dried Tomato & Feta Meatballs

Nutrition Facts

16 servings per container

Serving size

Amount Per Serving

Calories 70

% Daily Value*

Total Fat 5g	**6%**
Saturated Fat 0g	**0%**
Trans Fat 0g	
Cholesterol 40mg	**13%**
Sodium 70mg	**3%**
Total Carbohydrate 1g	**0%**
Dietary Fiber 0g	**0%**
Total Sugars 0g	
Includes 0g Added Sugars	**0%**
Protein 6g	**12%**
Vitamin D 0mcg	0%
Calcium 20mg	2%
Iron 0mg	0%
Potassium 90mg	2%
Vitamin A	2%
Magnesium	2%
Zinc	0%

*The % Daily Value (DV) tells you how much a nutrient in a serving of food contributes to a daily diet. 2,000 calories a day is used for general nutrition advice.

Recipe for making Sun-dried Tomato & Feta Meatballs
A low carbohydrate- & gluten-free Mediterranean-inspired meatball recipe
Serves: Sixteen (16) meatballs
Constituents

- One (1) lb. ground turkey.
- Quarter (¼) cup feta cheese, crumbled.
- Two (2) Tbl. (0.5 oz) sundried tomatoes, chopped.
- 1 Tbl. fresh thyme leaves (or ½ tablespoon dried thyme)
- One (1) egg
- Half (½) tablespoon garlic powder
- Quarter (¼) cup almond flour.
- Two (2) Tbl. water
- Olive oil (for frying).

Instructions

1. Mix all of the constituents (except olive oil) in a medium basin and blend well. Make 16 pieces of one (1) inch meatballs and get them fried in olive oil in a big sauce pan. Do not pack the meatballs or they wouldn't get brown & crisp - you might have to fry them in groups to get the paramount results. Cook for approx. 3 to 4 minutes, twist over and cook for an added 3 - 4 minutes or pending the time it becomes golden brown & cooked through. Take away from pan and put on paper towel-lined dish to soak up any added oil. These may be eaten unaided or dished up with marinara sauce & spaghetti squash for a complete meal.

Dessert

Two (2) squares Lindt 90 Percent Chocolate (See Table 12)

Day Five

(Totals: 1650 calories, 130g fat, 18g net carbohydrates, 80g protein)

Breakfast

- ✓ Two (2) Cream Cheese Pancakes (See Table 20 and figure 4)
- ✓ Two (2) pieces of cooked bacon (See Table 21)
- ✓ Coffee with two (2) tablespoons Heavy Cream (See Table 2)

Snack

- ✓ One (1) cup bone-broth (See Table 22)

Lunch

- ✓ Half (1/2) cup Anti-Pasta Salad (See Table 26 and figure 6)
- ✓ Four (4) Sundried Tomato & Feta Meatballs (See Table 27 and figure 7)

Snack

- ✓ Five (5) sticks of celery with Two (2) Tablespoons of Almond Butter (See Table 13)

Dinner

- ✓ One (1) cup of Cuban Pot Roast (See Table 28 and Figure 8)
- ✓ Two (2) cups of romaine lettuce, chopped (See Table 10)
- ✓ Two (2) Tablespoons of sour cream (See Table 29)
- ✓ One (1) Tablespoon of cilantro, chopped (optional)
- ✓ Quarter (1/4) cup of cheddar cheese, shredded (114 calories, 9g fat, .5g net carbohydrates, 7g protein).

Cuban Pot Roast (Taco-Salad Style)

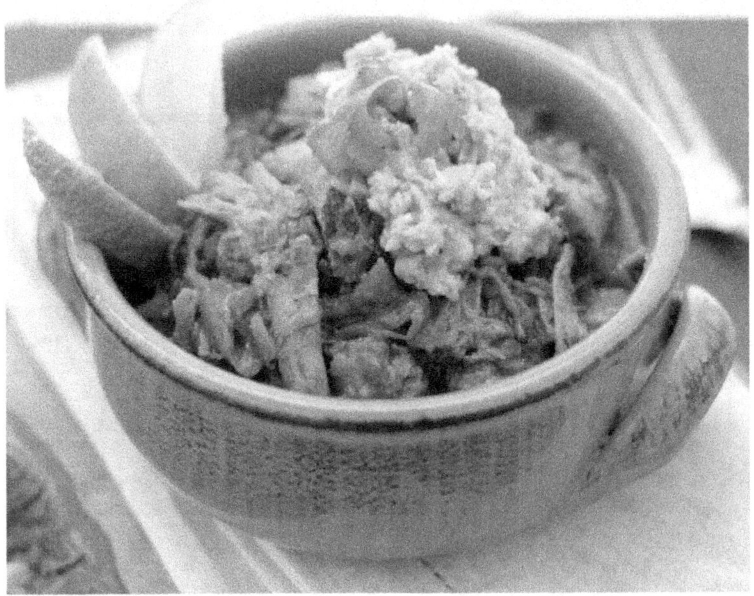

Fig. 8: Cuban Pot Roast Recipe – Low Carbohydrates and Gluten Free

Table 28. Nutritional facts for Cuban Pot Roast Recipe

Nutrition Facts

10 servings per container

Serving size

Amount Per Serving

Calories 30

	% Daily Value*
Total Fat 10g	**13%**
Saturated Fat 0g	**0%**
Trans Fat 0g	
Cholesterol 0mg	**0%**
Sodium 230mg	**10%**
Total Carbohydrate 6g	**2%**
Dietary Fiber 2g	**7%**
Total Sugars 2g	
Includes 0g Added Sugars	**0%**
Protein 1g	**2%**
Vitamin D 0mcg	0%
Calcium 50mg	4%
Iron 2mg	10%
Potassium 200mg	4%
Vitamin A	10%
Vitamin C	45%
Zinc	0%

*The % Daily Value (DV) tells you how much a nutrient in a serving of food contributes to a daily diet. 2,000 calories a day is used for general nutrition advice.

Recipe for making Cuban Pot Roast

A low carbohydrate Cuban Pot Roast recipe in the style of Ropa Vieja

Serves: Ten (10) servings

Ingredients

- Three (3) lb boneless chuck roast.
- Half (½) cup of salsa Verde.
- Half (½) cup of canned, chopped green chilies.
- One (1) cup of diced tomatoes.
- Two (2) Tablespoons of onion flakes, dried.
- One (1) tablespoon of garlic powder.
- Half (½) cup of red and yellow peppers sliced into strips.
- One (1) tablespoon of salt.
- Two (2) Tablespoons of ground cumin.
- One (1) tablespoon of ground coriander.
- One (1) tablespoon of dried oregano.
- One (1) tablespoon of chili powder.
- Half (½) tablespoon of black pepper.
- Two (2) tablespoons of apple cider vinegar.

Instructions

1. Munificently spice the roast with salt & pepper. Heat in a hot saucepan until all sides becomes brown. Put the meat in the base of a five (5) qt. crock pot. Include the chilies, salsa verde, & tomatoes to the saucepan you heated the meat in. Deglaze and get it boiled. Dispense over the meat you put in the crock pot. Include the garlic, onion flakes, salt, peppers, cumin, coriander, oregano, black pepper, chili powder, & apple cider vinegar, then stir. Cook for four 4 – 6 hours or until the meat becomes tender. Slice the meat & serve with toppings of your choice.

Two (2) Tablespoon Sour Cream

Table 29. Nutritional facts for (2) Tablespoon sour cream

Nutrition Facts

Serving size

Amount Per Serving

Calories 50

	% Daily Value*
Total Fat 5g	6%
Saturated Fat 0g	0%
Trans Fat 0g	
Sodium 0mg	0%
Total Carbohydrate 1g	0%
Dietary Fiber 0g	0%
Total Sugars 0g	
Includes 0g Added Sugars	0%
Protein 1g	2%

Not a significant source of cholesterol, vitamin D, calcium, iron, and potassium

*The % Daily Value (DV) tells you how much a nutrient in a serving of food contributes to a daily diet. 2,000 calories a day is used for general nutrition advice.

Quarter (1/4) Cup Shredded Cheddar Cheese

Table 30. Nutritional facts for 1/4 Cup Shredded Cheddar Cheese

Nutrition Facts

Serving size

Amount Per Serving

Calories 110

% Daily Value*

Total Fat 9g	**12%**
Saturated Fat 0g	**0%**
Trans Fat 0g	
Sodium 0mg	**0%**
Total Carbohydrate < 1g	**0%**
Dietary Fiber 0g	**0%**
Total Sugars 0g	
Includes 0g Added Sugars	**0%**
Protein 7g	**14%**

Not a significant source of cholesterol, vitamin D, calcium, iron, and potassium

*The % Daily Value (DV) tells you how much a nutrient in a serving of food contributes to a daily diet. 2,000 calories a day is used for general nutrition advice.

Dessert

- ✓ **Two (2) squares Lindt 90 percent Chocolate (See Table 12)**

Day Six

(Totals: 1600 calories, 120g fat, 19g net carbohydrates, 89g protein)

Breakfast

- ✓ **Three (3) eggs (scrambled or fried) (See Table 31)**

- ✓ **One (1) tablespoon butter (See Table 32)**

- ✓ **Two (20 pieces of cooked bacon (See Table 21)**

- ✓ **Coffee with two (2) tablespoons Heavy Cream (See Table 2)**

Three (3) eggs (scrambled or fried)

Table 31. Nutritional facts for 3 eggs (scrambled or fried)

Nutrition Facts

Serving size

Amount Per Serving

Calories 220

% Daily Value*

Total Fat 14g	**18%**
Saturated Fat 0g	**0%**
Trans Fat 0g	
Sodium 0mg	**0%**
Total Carbohydrate 1g	**0%**
Dietary Fiber 0g	**0%**
Total Sugars 0g	
Includes 0g Added Sugars	**0%**
Protein 19g	**38%**

Not a significant source of cholesterol, vitamin D, calcium, iron, and potassium

*The % Daily Value (DV) tells you how much a nutrient in a serving of food contributes to a daily diet. 2,000 calories a day is used for general nutrition advice.

One (1) Tablespoon butter

Table 32. Nutritional facts for 1 tablespoon butter

Nutrition Facts

Serving size

Amount Per Serving

Calories 35

	% Daily Value*
Total Fat 4g	**5%**
Saturated Fat 0g	**0%**
Trans Fat 0g	
Sodium 0mg	**0%**
Total Carbohydrate 0g	**0%**
Dietary Fiber 0g	**0%**
Total Sugars 0g	
Includes 0g Added Sugars	**0%**
Protein 0g	**0%**

Not a significant source of cholesterol, vitamin D, calcium, iron, and potassium

*The % Daily Value (DV) tells you how much a nutrient in a serving of food contributes to a daily diet. 2,000 calories a day is used for general nutrition advice.

✓ **Twenty-four (24) raw almonds**

Table 33. Nutritional facts for 24 raw almonds

Nutrition Facts

Serving size

Amount Per Serving
Calories 170

% Daily Value*

Total Fat 15g	**19%**
Saturated Fat 0g	**0%**
Trans Fat 0g	
Sodium 0mg	**0%**
Total Carbohydrate 2g	**1%**
Dietary Fiber 0g	**0%**
Total Sugars 0g	
Includes 0g Added Sugars	**0%**
Protein 6g	**12%**

Not a significant source of cholesterol, vitamin D, calcium, iron, and potassium

*The % Daily Value (DV) tells you how much a nutrient in a serving of food contributes to a daily diet. 2,000 calories a day is used for general nutrition advice.

Lunch

- ✓ One (1) cup of Cuban Pot Roast (See Table 28 and Figure 8)

- ✓ Two (2) cups of chopped romaine lettuce (See Table 10)

- ✓ Two (2) Tablespoon of sour cream (See Table 29)

- ✓ One (1) Tablespoon of chopped cilantro (optional)

- ✓ Quarter (1/4) cup of shredded cheddar cheese (See Table 29)

Snack

- ✓ One (1) cup of bone broth (See Table 22)

Dinner

- ✓ 1.5 cup of Chili-Spaghetti Squash Casserole (See Table 23 and Figure 5)

- ✓ Two (2) cups of raw baby spinach (See Table 24)

- ✓ One (1) Tablespoon of ranch dressing (sugar free) (See Table 25).

Dessert

- ✓ Two (2) square Lindt 90 percent Chocolate (See Table 12)

Day Seven

(Totals: 1600 calories, 130g fat, 20g net carbohydrates, 90g protein)

Breakfast

- ✓ Two (2) Cream-Cheese Pancakes (See Table 20 and figure 4)
- ✓ Two (2) pieces of bacon, cooked (See Table 21)
- ✓ Coffee with two (2) tablespoons Heavy Cream (See Table 2)

Snack

- ✓ Two (2) String Cheese (160 calories, 12g fat, 2g net carbs, 16g protein)

Lunch

- ✓ Half (1/2) cup of Anti-Pasta Salad (See Table 26 and figure 6)
- ✓ Four (4) Sundried Tomato & Feta Meatballs (See Table 27 and figure 7)

Snack

- ✓ One (1) of cup bone-broth (See Table 22)

Dinner

- ✓ One (1) cup of Cuban Pot Roast (See Table 28 and Figure 8)
- ✓ Two (2) cups of chopped romaine lettuce (See Table 10)
- ✓ Two (2) Tablespoon of sour cream (See Table 29)
- ✓ One (1) Tablespoon of chopped cilantro (optional)
- ✓ Quarter (1/4) cup of shredded cheddar cheese (See Table 29)

Dessert

- ✓ Two (2) squares Lindt 90 Percent Chocolate (See Table 12)

CHAPTER THREE

Eating Low Carbohydrate Meals Doesn't Mean Flavorless Diet Food

The greatest part of low carbohydrate meal is that you can still have highly nourishing, spicy foods – dieting is not actually a part of the way of life. Your body controls your appetite naturally, so maintaining low carbohydrate intakes is the main concern. Your ability to do that while still enjoying roast-fish and huge, healthy salads is what makes low carbohydrate meal very easy to get attached to, and get rid of excess weight for good.

www.ingramcontent.com/pod-product-compliance
Lightning Source LLC
Chambersburg PA
CBHW050851260726
48660CB00006B/2563